Managing Parkinson's

With Diet

Yuchi Yang, MS, RD

Table of Contents

Acknowledgments

I want to express my deepest appreciation to my clients for trusting me with their nutritional questions and concerns.

Disclaimer

The dietary approach listed in this book does not replace the other treatments prescribed by your physician and does not mean that you can now discontinue medications without first discussing the issue with your physician. The information provided in this book is general recommendations for individuals with Parkinson's disease. The information provided in this book should not be used for diagnosing purposes or be substituted for medical advice. As with any new or ongoing treatment, always consult your healthcare providers before beginning any new treatment including dietary modification.

The author provides resources, references, and website links for your information only. The author and American Nutrition Counseling, LLC are not responsible for the information, products or contents provided in these resources, references, and web sites.

Preface

I have been a registered dietitian for more than twenty years. The main reason that doctors refer their patients with Parkinson's disease (PD) to me is that they see a lot of fluctuation in their patients' response to medication with their diet, especially protein. As a registered dietitian, I help patients to estimate how much protein they need, to counsel them as such and provide advice on how to manage their diet to achieve a day-to-day consistency.

This book is not to replace dietary suggestions and treatments provided by your health care providers. It is my hope that this book will provide some dietary guidance to patients with Parkinson's and their friends and family members that care for these patients.

In chapter 2, you will find nutrition information and research findings on managing Parkinson's disease with diet. In chapter 3, I have listed step-by-step on how to design your own meal plan for patients with PD. In addition, I have included 14 healthy breakfasts, lunches, dinners, and snacks in Chapter 4. You can mix and match these meals and snacks to create your own weekly meal plan.

Research continues to explore the science behind diet and nutrition for the risks of Parkinson's and how to manage it. Further research and studies will result in even more compelling dietary recommendations. In the meantime, this book can be used as a guide to managing Parkinson's with diet.

Yuchi Yang, MS, RD
American Nutrition Counseling, LLC
www.anutritioncounseling.com

Chapter 1: Parkinson's Disease

Parkinson's disease (PD) is a disorder that affects part of the brain called substantia nigra. Symptoms generally develop slowly over years. Tremors are very common. It also causes stiffness or slowing of movement.

There are five stages of progression in Parkinson's disease. During Stage One, patients have mild symptoms that usually do not affect their daily activities. As PD progresses, movement control will become more challenging. In Stage Four and Five, patients need help with their daily activities.

Although there is no cure for Parkinson's disease yet, symptoms can be treated with medication. Levodopa, L-dopa, is the most commonly used drug for Parkinson's disease.

Possible Risk Factors

There are genetic and environmental factors that increase the risks of Parkinson's disease (PD). Studies have indicated that environmental toxins important in PD include pesticides, herbicides, and heavy metals.

Eating behaviors have also shown some associations in PD studies. Increased iron intake could cause higher oxidation. High iron diet may be associated with the increased risk of PD in certain population.

Higher consumption of milk and dairy products has increased PD risk.

Patients with PD had lower intake of polyunsaturated fats, higher intake of saturated fats, a higher intake of carbohydrates, lower protein, and low in certain nutrients such as folate. Patients with PD also had lower bone mass index and lower vitamin D and vitamin E levels.

Excitotoxins are toxins that excite the brain and nerve cells beyond their normal physiologic capacity. Excitotoxins such as aspartame and monosodium glutamate (MSG) overstimulate neuron receptors, affect brain cells and promote neuronal death.

Although we cannot control our genetic factors, we can make some positive environmental and behavior changes to reduce the risks of Parkinson's disease.

Behaviors that may Decrease the Risk

Eat Good Fats

Studies have shown some behaviors might have some protective effects in PD. Polyunsaturated fats intake was associated with lower PD risk, and dietary fats modified the association of PD risk with pesticide exposure. Higher omega-3 fats intake has shown to reduce the risk of PD.

Drink Tea and/or Coffee

Studies have found that people who drink coffee or tea tend to have a lower risk of having Parkinson's disease. A Japanese study has shown that people with the highest consumption of tea associated with more than 60% lower risk of developing PD compared with the lowest consumption group.

Eat Fruits, Vegetables, and Legumes

Studies also found a protective effect of beta-carotene (beta carotene can be found in carrots) in PD in a Japanese population. Eating legumes was also found protective. Higher vitamin E intake has shown decreased risk of PD. Eating phytonutrients rich foods such as strawberries and blueberries have shown to reduce PD risk.

Get Adequate Amount of Vitamin D

Studies have suggested that eating adequate vitamin D in the diet, or taking a Vitamin D supplement was associated with a lower risk of developing PD. In a Finland study, people with the highest serum vitamin D had a 67% reduced risk of PD compared with people with the lowest serum vitamin D levels.

Avoid Excitotoxins

Excitotoxins such as aspartame and monosodium glutamate (MSG) overstimulate neuron receptors, affect brain cells and promote neuronal death. Whenever buying processed foods, it is recommended to read the ingredient lists and avoid artificial sweeteners and MSG.

When eating out, try to avoid MSG as much as possible. Nowadays, most of the restaurants are very accommodating to customers' requests. When eating out, you can request no MSG added to your dishes.

Chapter 2: Managing Parkinson's with Diet

Eat Healthfully, but Not Too Much

Americans eat an average of over 3,000 calories a day which is much higher than the recommended amount. Overweight in midlife has been associated with the increased risk for Parkinson's disease (PD). People with Body Mass Index (BMI) of 30 (i.e. obese) had twice the risk of developing PD than those with a BMI of lower than 23.

In studies, lower calorie diets seemed to slow down the PD's progression. In animal studies, dietary restriction has been found to reduce the destruction of dopamine producing brain cells.

Based on these findings, it is a good idea to eat healthfully, but not too much. For most men, the recommended intake is between 2,000 – 2,400 calories a day and for most women, the suggested amount is between 1,600 - 2,000 calories a day. As a registered dietitian, when I work with patients with PD to develop their personal meal plans, I usually have 300-500 calories for breakfasts, and 300-500 calories for lunches, and 500-800 calories for dinners. If they need 1-3 snacks during the day, I often suggest snacks that have 100-200 calories for each snack. In next page, you will find an example of a healthful daily meal plan for 1,660 calories. To find out your specific caloric needs, please consult a registered dietitian.

Below is An Example of One Day Healthful Menu

Meals & Snacks	Food Items	Calories
Breakfast	1 cup Cheerios, 1 cup almond milk, 1 orange, 12 almonds	350
Lunch	1 avocado sushi roll (6 pieces), 1 miso soup, 1 apple, 6 cashews	450
Dinner	1 cup brown rice, 1 cup cooked kidney beans, 3 oz. ground pork, 1 cup green beans, 1 tsp. olive oil	600
Snack 1	1 pear	100
Snack 2	1 oz. coconut chips	160
Total		1,660

Malnutrition

Patients with Parkinson's disease have been found to be at greater risks for malnutrition. Malnutrition includes not getting enough calories, protein, and nutrients that are needed for health and well-being.

Studies have shown that people with PD were four times more likely to have a weight loss of 10 lbs. or more. When I conduct nutrition assessments of patients with PD, I always record their current weight as well as their previous weight. This will give me a better picture of their nutritional status.

Weight loss is common in patients with PD. There are many factors may contribute to weight loss. First, they may have decreased food intake as a result of Dysphagia (difficulty swallowing), poor appetite due to depression, anxiety, and food restriction because food "turned off" the levodopa effect. Second, they may have increased energy expenditure resulting from hyperkinetic movements (tremor).

It is important to monitor patients' weight on a regular basis and adjust their meal plan as needed. One of my patients with PD has a body mass index (BMI) of 20 which is within a normal range. However, when I asked her how much was her weight before? I realized that she had lost 15 lbs. since she was diagnosed with PD. To prevent malnutrition and further weight loss, I have helped her to develop a meal plan that consists of few hundred more calories and more nutrients than her current food intake.

No More Low-Fat Diets

About 60% of the brain is fats. Our brain requires essential fats in order to function properly. Americans have been ingrained with low-fat messages for the past few decades. I have seen clients with Parkinson's disease eating low-fat diets for years. The first dietary suggestion that I gave them is to increase good fats in their diet.

How Much Oil Do You Need?

Oils and fats are essential nutrients to our brain and they also add flavors to our dishes. Eating adequate amount of oils and fats is essential for our health.

I recommend 35% of calories coming from oils and fats. For most people with Parkinson's disease, this is equivalent to 5 - 7 teaspoons per meal and 1-3 teaspoons for all of the daily snacks combined.

For some of you who are interested in the numbers. Here is how I came up with the numbers. For a 2,000 calorie diet:

2,000 x 35% = 700 calories from fat

1 gram of fat has 9 calories, so

$700 \div 9 \approx 78$ grams of fat

1 teaspoon of fat has about 5 grams.

$78 \div 5 \approx 16$ teaspoons of fat a day

In summary, for a 2,000 calorie diet, you can have five teaspoons of fat each meal and 1-3 teaspoons of fat for all snacks combined.

Now, let's look at the following breakfast:

1 cup oatmeal cooked (in water)
1 cup skim milk
1 orange

Is this a healthy breakfast? My answer is no. This breakfast has close to zero fat. Let's make this breakfast healthier by adding some oils and fats.

By including 1 cup coconut milk, 6 almonds and ½ avocados, we have added some healthy fats. Here is one healthy breakfast for patients with Parkinson's:

1 cup oatmeal cooked (in water)
1 cup coconut milk
6 almonds
½ avocado

Fat Contents of Common Foods

Items/Fat amount	1 tsp. fat*	2 tsp.*	3 tsp.*
Olive oil	1 tsp.		
Butter or mayo	½ tbsp.	1 tbsp.	
Dressing or cream cheese or gravy or coconut milk	1 tbsp.	2 tbsp.	3 tbsp.
Cheese (1 oz. part skim = 1 fat)	1 oz. feta	1 oz. cheddar	
Avocado (large)	1/6	1/3	½
Peanut butter	2/3 tbsp.		2 tbsp.
Almonds	1 tbsp.	2 tbsp.	3 tbsp.
Guacamole	2 tbsp.	4 tbsp.	8 tbsp.
Bacon	1 slice	2 slices	
Hummus	4 tbsp.	8 tbsp.	12 tbsp.
Salmon	3 oz.	6 oz.	
Ground beef (90% lean)		3 oz.	
Ground beef (80% lean)			3 oz.
Pork chops		3-4 oz.	
Egg (large)	1	2	
Olives (large)	8 olives		
2% milk	1 cup	2 cups	

*Please note that these are approximate numbers for easy calculations; therefore, you can apply the information on a daily basis. For more precise numbers, please visit the USDA National Nutrient Database.

How Much Fat Do You Eat in One Meal?

You can use the previous table to figure out how much fat you consume in one meal.

For example, if you have the following dinner:

1 cup brown rice (no fat)
6 oz. salmon (2 tsp. oil)
1 tbsp. olive oil for cooking (3 tsp. oil)
1 cup broccoli
16 oz. water (no fat)

The total amount of fat for this dinner is 5 tsp. This is a healthy and delicious dinner that you can enjoy often.

Note: 1 tablespoon (tbsp.) equals 3 teaspoons (tsp.).

Different Types of Oils and Fats

There are three different categories of fats and oils based on their chemical structures:

1. **Polyunsaturated fatty acids (PUFA)**
    They have more than one unsaturated carbon bond in the molecule. Common sources include soybean oil, fish oil, and nuts.
    Nuts and seeds, and fish oil have shown to reduce the rate of Parkinson's progression.

2. **Monounsaturated fatty acids (MUFA)**
    They have one unsaturated carbon bond. Olive oil, avocados, and macadamia nuts are good sources of monounsaturated fats.
    Olive oil has been associated with reduced PD progression.

3. **Saturated fats**
    They have no double bonds. They are solid at room temperature. Butter, meat fats, and coconut oil are saturated fats.
    Coconut oil was associated with the reduced PD progression.

Studies have shown that MUFAs and PUFAs suggested decreased PD progression while saturated fats from animal source may worsen the condition.

Omega-3 Fats

The main essential fats in the diet are polyunsaturated fats. Polyunsaturated fats include omega-3 fats and omega-6 fats.

Omega-3 fats have been associated with reduced PD progression.

Common sources of omega-3 fats: salmon, walnuts, flax seeds, and chia seeds

Common sources of omega-6 fats: sunflower oil, soybean oil, and corn oil

A good ratio of omega-3 fat to omega-6 fat intake is about 1:1. However, in a typical American diet, the ratio is 1:15. In other words, most Americans consume too much omega-6 fats compared to omega-3 fats. The imbalances of fats have been linked to many health problems.

Tips on how to increase omega-3 fats in your diet:

- Eat 1 ounce of nuts or seeds daily.
- Eat fish twice to three times a week.

If you choose to take fish oil supplements, I recommend 1,200-2,400 mg daily. But, if you are taking medications, please talk with your doctor before starting on fish oil supplements. It's because fish oil supplements may interact with some medications.

Eating a Balance of Fats

Consuming different types of oils and fats is essential for brain health. A typical American diet usually is high in saturated fats and low in monounsaturated fats and omega-3 fats. Below are some tips to help you achieve a better ratio of different fats:

- Cook with olive oil.
- Eat one ounce of nuts or seeds daily.
- Enjoy avocado.
- Have fish twice to three times a week.
- Cut off obvious meat fats and skins. (Studies have suggested an association of the increased Parkinson's disease risk with high animal fat intake.)

Eating a good ratio of different fats in the right amount can be easy. Below is an example of a one-day fat intake from different food items:

- 6 oz. fish (2 tsp. fat)
- 2 tsp. coconut oil (2 tsp. fat)
- 1 oz. almonds (3 tsp. fat)
- 6 tsp. olive oil for cooking or dressing (6 tsp. fat)
- ½ large avocado (3 tsp. fat)

Total fat from the food items above is 16 tsp. and includes saturated fats, monounsaturated fats, and polyunsaturated fats.

Levodopa and Dietary Protein Competition

Levodopa (L-dopa) is prescribed by the doctor to treat the symptoms of Parkinson's disease. Parkinson's symptoms include tremors, stiffness, and slowness of movement. These symptoms are caused by a lack of dopamine in the brain. Dopamine in the brain controls and regulates our movement. PD drug, Levodopa, works by being converted to dopamine in the brain, which improves the motor functions of patients with PD.

Amino acids are building blocks of proteins. L-dopa is a large amino acid. Dietary protein may compete with L-dopa in the intestines for absorption. In addition, dietary protein is broken down to amino acids and be absorbed into the body. These amino acids can compete with L-dopa to cross the blood-brain barrier and decrease the efficacy of the drug. Such problem of protein and levodopa competition usually appears years after the initiation of L-dopa therapy.

There are some interventions that have been suggested to ameliorate motor functions. First, take medication one hour prior to the meal. This will reduce the impact of dietary protein and PD medication competition and increase the efficacy of the medication.

Second, consume smaller amount of protein at breakfast and lunch. This allows more L-dopa entering to the brain and will improve the motor function during the day.

Third, eat more protein at dinner and evening. This will help to assure adequate protein intake and prevent malnutrition.

Studies have shown that high protein diet decreased mobility in patients who are taking L-dopa. Based on this finding, there are two suggestions:

- "protein restriction diet"
- "protein redistribution diet".

The original "protein-redistribution diet" is limited to 7 grams of protein before the evening meal, and is unrestricted protein afterwards until bedtime. This will maximize daytime motor function. However, limiting to 7 grams of protein may not be a feasible nor acceptable option for many patients with PD. When I help my patients with PD to develop their meal plan, one of the goals is to have less than half protein during the day and more than half (about 30 grams or more) protein for dinner and evening. A meal plan like this will help to improve their daytime motor function while honoring their food preference and habits.

Below is one example of a meal plan and medication schedule:

7 am: PD medication

8 am: Breakfast:
- 1 cup coconut milk
- 6 crackers
- ½ medium avocado

- 1 cup grapes
- 12 almonds

11 am: PD medication

Noon: Lunch:
- 1 cup rice
- 1 cup stir-fry Napa cabbage (with 1 tbsp. olive oil)
- 1 cup stir-fry onions with kidney beans (½ cup onions, ½ cup kidney beans, 1 tsp. coconut oil)
- 1 cup strawberries

4 pm: PD medication

5 pm: Dinner:
- 1 cup soy milk
- 3 oz. salmon
- 2 cup salad with 2 tbsp. dressing
- 1 medium potato
- ½ cup blueberries

9 pm: PD medication

10 pm: Snack: 12 cashews

This one-day meal plan provides about 1,600 calories and 57 grams protein. This meal plan may meet the nutritional needs of an elderly woman with a healthy weight. For your specific nutritional needs, please consult a registered dietitian or your physician.

Men usually need more calories and dietary protein than women. You can modify the above meal plan by replacing the night time snack of 12 cashews with a peanut butter and jelly sandwich. This replacement will provide 400 extra calories and additional 8 grams of protein.

Get Adequate Protein, but Not Too Much

As noted in the previous section, dietary protein competes with L-dopa and affects the efficacy of L-dopa; therefore, it is not a good idea to eat too much protein. Studies have reported that a daily protein intake of about 1.6 grams per kilogram of body weight was likely to diminish L-dopa efficacy in PD patients with motor fluctuations. In addition, studies have correlated excessive protein intake with PD progression.

Most Americans eat about 100 grams of protein per day, which is more than the recommended daily amount (RDA) of 0.8 grams per kilogram of body weight. The following table shows the daily protein recommendations for adults.

Daily Protein Recommendations for Adult Men and Women

Protein/Gender	Adult Men	Adult Women
Protein (g)	56	46
Protein % calories	10-35%	10-35%

Source: Dietary Guidelines 2015-2020 Recommendations and Institute of Medicine. Dietary Reference Intakes: The essential guide to nutrient requirements. Washington (DC): The National Academies Press; 2006.

The elderly patients with PD may need more than current RDA to maintain physical function and optimal health.

When I work with patients with PD, I usually start with 0.8 g/kg body weight while monitoring their weight.

For example, a man with a body weight of 180 lbs., his RDA for protein will be 66 grams per day. This is how I calculate it:

180 lb. divided by 2.2 equals to 82 kilograms.

82 kilograms multiply by 0.8 equals to 66 grams per day.

Weight loss is a common concern among patients with PD. If a patient with PD has failed to maintain his or her body weight and/or lean muscle mass with the recommended daily amount of protein, I will increase the dietary protein from 0.8 g/kg body weight to 1.0 g/kg body weight.

Eat Less Dairy Products

Many Americans consume a lot of milk and dairy products. Studies have suggested an association between the increased incidences of Parkinson's disease (PD) with the excessive consumption of dairy products. Dairy products were also found to be associated with more rapid PD progression.

Milk and Dairy products contains a lot of protein. Each serving has 8 grams of protein. Dietary protein competes with PD drug, Levodopa. Therefore, patients with PD need to control their protein intake throughout their day.

There was a man in his 60s, coming to my office to get some help to manage his Parkinson's disease with diet. I helped him to develop a meal plan that would assist him to achieve a day-to-day consistency. During the nutrition session, I found that he often had five servings of milk and dairy products a day. Based on the study findings noted earlier, I advised him to limit his dairy products to one serving a day.

Soybeans

Soybeans contain all of the essential amino acids. That is they have a complete protein. Soybeans have been grown and harvested for thousands of years. They are important protein sources for many people in certain regions.

There are plenty of studies done on soybeans. Many showed conflicting conclusions on various health conditions. For patients with Parkinson's disease (PD), soybeans have shown favorable effects on the motor functions. Study results indicated that soy partly increased the bioavailability of PD medication, levodopa.

If my patients would like to have soybeans in their diet, I encourage them to have Edamame (green soybeans), soybean milk or tofu and avoid highly processed soy protein powder or vegan patty that contains soy protein isolates.

Have an Adequate Amount of Fiber

Dietary Fiber

Dietary fibers are carbohydrates and lignin that cannot be digested by humans. It can be found in whole grains, beans, fruits, and vegetables. Dietary fiber increases L-dopa absorption with higher blood concentration. In other words, dietary fiber increases the bioavailability of Parkinson's drug, L-dopa. It also helps bowel movement and prevents constipation which is a common problem among people with Parkinson's. Therefore, it is important to eat an adequate amount of dietary fiber.

The average fiber intake in the U.S. is only 17 grams a day which is way below the suggested amount by the Institute of Medicine.

Daily Adequate Intake for Fiber Set by the Institute of Medicine: 14 Grams per 1,000 Calories

For most adults, this translates to 28-35 grams a day.

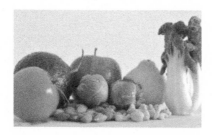

Dietary Fiber Contents of Common Foods

Food	Portion Size	Fiber per Portion (g)*
Beans (black, kidney)	½ cup cooked	6–9
Green peas, cooked	½ cup	4
Whole-wheat English muffin	1 muffin	4
Raspberries, blackberries	½ cup	4
Sweet potato with skin	1 medium	4
Shredded wheat cereal	1 oz.	4
Avocado	½ medium	4
Apple or pear with skin	1 small	4
Greens (spinach), cooked	½ cup	3
Nuts (Almonds)	1 ounce	3
Whole wheat spaghetti	½ cup cooked	3
Banana	1 medium	3
Orange	1 medium	3
Potato with skin	1 small	3
Winter squash, cooked	½ cup	3
Tomato paste	¼ cup	3
Broccoli, cooked	½ cup	3
Quinoa	½ cup	2.5
Brown Rice	½ cup	2
Strawberries	½ cup	2
Grapes, red or green	½ cup	1

*Please note that these are approximate numbers for easy calculations. For more precise numbers, please visit the USDA National Nutrient Database.

How Much Dietary Fiber Do You Eat?

You can refer back to the previous table to figure out how much dietary fiber you have for one meal.

Below is an example of breakfast:

- 1 cup shredded wheat (4 grams fiber)
- 1 cup coconut milk (no fiber)
- 6 almonds (1 grams fiber)
- 1 orange (3 grams fiber)

The total amount of fiber for this breakfast is 8 grams. This is a healthy and delicious meal with adequate amount of fiber that you can enjoy often.

Tally Your Fiber Consumption

Use the form below to see how much dietary fiber in your diet.

Meals & Snacks	Food Items	Fiber (grams)
Breakfast		
Lunch		
Dinner		
Snack 1		
Snack 2		
Snack 3		
Total		

Tips on How to Increase Your Dietary Fiber

It is wise to increase dietary fiber gradually to prevent any gastrointestinal discomfort. I suggest that you increase the fiber intake by 5 grams each week until you reach the goal of 30 grams a day.

For example, if your current fiber consumption is 15 grams a day. You will increase your fiber intake to 20 grams in the first week. In the second week, your goal will be 25 grams a day. Repeat the same process and you will reach your goal of 30 grams by the third week.

There are many ways that you can incorporate in your diet to add additional 5 grams of fiber. Here are some examples:

- Choose whole wheat sandwiches instead of white bread. (about 5 grams)
- Add a cup of veggie to dinner. (6 grams)
- Eat a medium size apple. (5-6 grams)
- Eat ½ cup cooked beans. (6-9 grams)

By tallying your fiber consumption once a week, you can identify the high fiber food items that you can add to your diet. This process will help you stay focused and attain the goal of 30 grams of fiber a day.

Because fiber absorbs water, you may need to increase your water intake. It is a good idea to carry a water bottle with you so you can drink throughout the day.

Daily Liquid Goals Set by the Institute of Medicine:

- **15 cups a day for men (18 years of age or older)**
- **11 cups a day for women (18 years of age or older)**

Liquids include water, soup, beverages, yogurt, applesauce, and more.

One Day Menu with 33 Grams of Fiber

Meals & Snacks	Food Items	Fiber (grams)
Breakfast	1 cup oatmeal, 1 cup coconut milk, 1 orange, 12 cashews	11
Lunch	1 peanut butter sandwiches (2 whole wheat bread, 1 tbsp. peanut butter), 1 apple, 1 cup water	9
Dinner	1 medium sweet potato, 6 oz. salmon, ½ cup broccoli, 1 tbsp. olive oil, 1 cup water	7
Snack 1	½ cup blueberries	4
Snack 2	1 small avocado	2
Total		33

This one day menu has 1,800 calories and 33 grams of dietary fiber.

Eat Fresh Fruits & Vegetables

High intakes of fruits and vegetables were found to be associated with the lower risk of developing Parkinson's disease (PD). Phytonutrients in fresh fruits and vegetables were also suggested to reduce PD progression. On the other hand, canned fruits and vegetables were found to be associated with more rapid PD progression. Bisphenol A (BPA) in the inner coating of food cans and aluminum content of the cans were suggested for the increased PD progression. Thus it is important to eat fresh fruits and vegetables instead of canned fruits and vegetables.

Dark leafy green vegetables like kale, collard greens, and spinach and fruits such as blueberries and raspberries have shown some beneficial effects.

Organic produce, free of pesticides, with higher nutrient contents than its conventional counterpart are healthier choices for patients with PD. However, the cost can be much higher. The alternative is to buy the produce that is likely to have the fewest pesticide residues such as banana, papaya, cabbage, kiwi, oranges, pineapples, avocado, and onions.

The daily recommended vegetables intake is 2-4 cups. However, the average American consumption is much lower than the recommended amount. When clients walking into my office, telling me that "I don't like vegetables. I know I suppose to eat some vegetables but please don't tell me to eat vegetables because they don't taste good." For people like that, I usually ask them to try the following recipe, stir-fry Napa cabbage.

Stir-Fry Napa Cabbage

I have shared this recipe with a lot of people. Many of them have tried and really enjoyed it. It's very simply and very healthy.

- You can usually find Napa cabbage sitting next to green cabbage in a super market. You can slice it in the middle and put half back in the refrigerator for next time.
- Rinse half of Napa cabbage that you are going to cook under the water and shake off the water.
- Chop Napa cabbage into pieces.
- Snap a clove or two garlics and chop it small.
- Heat two tablespoons of original olive oil in the cooking pot, add garlic and a little bit of salt for taste. Stir fry garlic for twenty or thirty seconds so the flavor will come out.
- Add the chopped Napa cabbage into the pot. Stir fry to mix it well. Then cover the lid for about a minute or two. Then open up the lid, stir fry it a little bit so it won't get burned.
- When Napa cabbage gets softer, some of the water will come out. If your heat is high and water dries out. Then you will need to add one or two tablespoons of water. Stir fry it and cover it. Repeat this for few times until Napa cabbage is cooked through and turns soft. It will take about 5 minutes.

Studies have shown that some people have more sensitive taste buds; they can taste the bitterness of the vegetables. By adding oil, garlics, and salt to stir fry vegetables, the bitterness will decrease.

You can use this method to stir fry other vegetables like broccoli and cauliflower.

Plant-Based Diet

A plant-based diet or vegan diet is a way of eating that excludes all animal sources. Studies have shown that plant-based diet may decrease the risk of PD and also slow down the PD progression. A plant-based diet contains less protein, thus increase L-dopa efficacy. In addition, a plant-based diet has more fiber contents which will help with the management of PD.

A healthy plant-based diet consists of 10-15% of total calories from protein. This diet can be combined with the "protein redistribution diet" with the main protein intake concentrated at dinner and night time snack. This dietary approach will help patients to manage their Parkinson's.

Protein-rich plant foods include legumes, nuts, seeds, and soybeans. Grains such as quinoa, rice, and wheat also contain some protein.

Vitamin B12 is generally found in all animal sources. Vitamin B12 protects the nervous system. Without vitamin B12, permanent damage can result. Fatigue and numbness and tingling in the hands or feet are some of the early signs.

Gastric acid helps us to absorb vitamin B12. As we age, our stomachs produce less gastric acid. Thus, it reduces the body's ability to absorb vitamin B12. The U.S. Food and Drug Administration set the Daily Value (DV) for vitamin B-12 at 6 micrograms. If you are on a vegan diet, to prevent vitamin B12 deficiencies, consider taking a vitamin B12 supplement.

Below is one example of a healthy plant-based meal plan for patients with Parkinson's disease:

Breakfast:
- 1 cup mung bean soup (½ cup bean, ½ cup water, 1 tbsp. sugar)
- 1 avocado
- 1 orange

Lunch:
- 1 bean avocado burrito
- 1 cup salad with 1 tbsp. dressing
- 1 cup strawberries

Afternoon snack:
- 1 apple

Dinner:
- 1 cup brown rice
- 6 oz. tofu
- 12 cashews
- 1 cup broccoli
- 1 tbsp. olive oil for cooking

Night time snack:
- 1 cup coconut milk

This meal plan has about 1,600 calories, 170 grams carbs, 50 grams protein, and 35 grams of fiber. This meal plan will meet the nutritional needs of an elderly woman with a body weight of 120 lbs.

Alleviate Constipation

Constipation is a common problem among patients with Parkinson's disease (PD). To alleviate constipation, here are the dietary suggestions:

Eat adequate amount of dietary fiber. Start with a minimum of 5 grams of dietary fibers in each meal. And increase the daily amount gradually to 25 grams for women and 35 grams for men. High-fiber foods include beans, fruits, vegetables, whole grains, nuts, and seeds.

Drink enough water and fluid. Gradually increase the total fluid consumption. The goal fluid intake for women is about 8-10 cups and for men is about 10-12 cups.

Consume adequate amount of good fats. Fats function as lubricants and will help to alleviate constipation. Coconut oil tends to speed up bowel movement and soften the stools. Some people may experience gastrointestinal discomfort with coconut oil consumption. When you start to incorporate coconut oil into your diet, it is prudent to start with a small amount like 1 teaspoon and gradually increase the amount as tolerated to 1-2 tbsp. a day.

The reasonable total daily fats intake for patients with Parkinson's disease is about 35% calories. For many people, this translates to about 16 tsp. of oil per day. To assure overall health and well-being, some of these dietary fat intakes have to come from essential fats, i.e. polyunsaturated fats.

Carbohydrates and Protein Ratio

Dietary protein raises blood large neutral amino acid (LNAA). Blood LNAA competes with PD drug, levodopa, to pass the blood-brain barrier. Thus, strict dietary protein (less than 7 grams) during daytime has been suggested to maximize the L-dopa efficacy. However, such protein restriction is difficult to comply with and may result in protein malnutrition.

A higher carbohydrate (carb) diet raises blood insulin, reduces blood LNAA, and increases the ratio of L-dopa to LNAA. Several studies have reported that diets with stable higher carbs to protein ratios such as 5:1 or 7:1 have lowered blood LNAA, thus improved motor functions. These findings suggested that a stringent daytime protein restriction (less than 7 grams) might not be necessary. In addition, an approach like this allows more protein intake during daytime and it is much easier for patients with PD to comply with than the protein restricted diet.

Meal plans and recipes included in this book are developed for patients with PD who are taking L-Dopa. These meal plans are created by the author based on the following study findings:

- "low protein diet (about RDA protein)"
- "protein redistribution diet"
- "carbohydrate-to-protein ratios".

These meal plans and recipes are general dietary suggestions for patients with Parkinson's disease. Due to the high carbohydrate contents of these meal plans and recipes, they are not appropriate for patients who have diabetes. Please consult your physician before starting any dietary interventions including the meal plans listed in this book.

The meal plan below has a carbohydrate-to-protein ratio of 5:1.

Breakfast:
- 1 bean avocado burrito (½ cup bean, ½ avocado, 1 wrap)
- 1 large apple
- 1 cup green tea

Lunch:
- 2 ½ cups pasta (2 cups pasta noodle, ½ cup pasta sauce, 5 tsp. olive oil)
- 3 oz. banana chips
- 1 cup dark coffee (If you like, you can add some coconut milk and/or sugar.)

Dinner:
- 1 cup soy milk (1 tbsp. sugar)
- 3 oz. pan-fry salmon
- 1 cup stir-fry broccoli (1tbsp. oil)
- 2 cups rice

This one-day meal plan has about 2,300 calories, 260 grams of carbs and 52 grams protein. The carbohydrate-to-protein ratio for this meal plan is 5:1 (260 ÷ 52 = 5:1).

Supplements

Please consult with your doctor before taking any supplements. As with any new or ongoing treatment, always consult your healthcare providers before beginning any new treatment including dietary supplements.

Supplementation with antioxidants has been suggested to reduce PD progression. However, this theory has not been proven.

Coenzyme Q10 (CoQ10) is one antioxidant that has been studied. Patients with PD often have reduced CoQ10 levels. Supplementation with CoQ10 was associated with the reduce PD progression.

Fish oil is a good source of omega -3 fats. Taking fish oil supplement was associated with improvements in depression among patients with PD.

CoQ10, fish oil, and vitamin D are potential topics that need further research. At this time, not enough is known to make specific recommendations.

On the other hand, high iron consumption has been associated with PD progression. Because iron is often included in multivitamins, patients with PD should avoid multivitamin mineral supplements containing iron, unless it is prescribed by their physician to treat iron–deficiency anemia.

Dietary Management of Dysphagia

Dysphagia is a condition with a difficulty in swallowing. Swallowing is a very complex process. Dysphagia can be caused by various reasons. Parkinson's disease is a gradually progressive, degenerative neurological disorder that impairs the patient's motor skills. Dysphagia is a common problem among patients with PD.

Symptoms of dysphagia may include coughing or gagging during eating, drooling, heartburn, and difficulty controlling food in the mouth. Patients may feel "food stuck in the throat or chest".

Dysphagia may decrease patients' total food intake and result in malnutrition and weight loss. Dysphagia also affects patients' ability to drink adequate amount of fluid, this may lead to dehydration.

PD Patients with Dysphagia may respond well to PD medication (L-dopa), feeding therapy, and/or procedures. Some foods and liquids are easier to swallow than others. Consistency and texture of food are also important things to consider. Commercial food thickeners, such as Thick-It and Thick and Easy, can help to improve patients' eating experience and total food intake. These products can be used to achieve desired consistency in pureed foods and beverages.

When dysphagia occurs, it is important to assess patients' total food and fluid intake. If Dysphagia symptoms are present over a long period of time, patients may lose weight and become malnourished. Dehydration can occur if there is difficulty swallowing liquids.

Dietary interventions of Dysphagia often involve making a change in the foods eaten and/or the consistency of food. If the total food intake decreases, one of the dietary intervention focuses will be to increase the caloric density of food. Small frequent meals may also help to increase the total food and fluid intake. If patients are unable to eat and drink enough by mouth, tube feedings may be needed.

Ketogenic Diet

Ketogenic diet is a high-fat, low-carbohydrate, and moderate protein diet. This diet forces the body to use fat instead of glucose. This will cause a rise in ketone bodies, which are byproducts of breakdown of fat. Ketones are alternative energy for brain neurons.

The ketogenic diet has been used at hospitals and medical clinics for decades for the treatment of epilepsy. One study tested the effects of the ketogenic diet on symptoms of Parkinson's disease. After 28 days on the ketogenic diet, these patients with PD have reported improvement in symptoms. However, some experienced adverse effects such as gastrointestinal (GI) discomfort, headache, increased irritability, and thirst.

There are several versions of ketogenic diets: classic ketogenic diet, modified Atkins diet, low glycemic index diet, and medium-chain triglyceride diet. These diets do not equal to starvation. Instead, they are precisely calculated to meet the nutritional needs of patients while forcing the body to produce ketones.

The classic ketogenic diet is based on a ratio of grams of fat to combined grams of carbohydrate and protein of 3:1 or 4:1. While Modified Atkins diet, Low glycemic index, and MCT diets are usually have a ratio of 2:1 or 1:1.

Below is one example of a ketogenic meal plan with an approximate ratio of 2.6:1:

Breakfast:

- 1 cup coffee with 1 tbsp. coconut oil
- One cup salad (1 cup lettuce, 4 olives, ¼ avocado, 1 tbsp. extra virgin olive oil, black pepper, salt)
- 1 scrambled eggs (one egg, 1 tbsp. olive oil)

Lunch:

- Zucchini pasta (1 zucchini, 1 tbsp. coconut oil, 1 tbsp. extra virgin olive oil, ½ cup pasta sauce)
- ½ avocado

Dinner:

- 6 oz. pan-fry salmon (1 tbsp. coconut oil &1 tbsp. olive oil for pan fry)
- ¼ cup butternut squash (1 tbsp. extra virgin olive oil)
- 1 cup broccoli (1 tbsp. olive oil)

This one-day meal plan has about 1,900 calories, 180 grams fat, 46 grams protein, and 22 grams net carbohydrates (carbs).

This is how you calculate net carbohydrates:

Total Carbs – Dietary Fiber = Net Carbs

The classic ketogenic diet has about 10 grams net carbs, 10% calories from protein and more than 85% calories from fats. Medium-chain triglycerides (MCT) ketogenic diet has about 15% energy from carbs, 10% from protein, 30% from long-chain fats, and 45% from MCT oil.

Ketogenic diet is a form of Medical Nutrition Therapy. Patients need to consult their physician before the initiation of ketogenic diet. Patients with certain conditions such as gastrointestinal problems, kidney problems, or liver problems may not be good candidates for ketogenic diet. The ketogenic diet usually starts at a lower ratio (fat: protein and carbs) and gradually increases to the target ratio over 1-2 weeks as tolerated. In addition, patients need to be closely monitored by their physician for any adverse reactions once they start on the ketogenic diet.

Everyone Has Unique Dietary Needs

Parkinson's disease (PD) is a chronic and progressive movement disorder. There are five stages of PD starting with mild to severe symptoms. Dietary needs and interventions will be different for different stages. At the initial stage, the nutritional needs and interventions will be similar to the ones without PD for the same gender and age group. The focus will be healthy eating pattern with an emphasis on not eating excessive energy and eating good fats and plenty of legumes, fresh fruits, and vegetables.

As the PD progresses and tremor worsens, patients with PD may start losing weight. It is important to modify the meal plan at the first sign of weight loss to prevent malnutrition.

When dysphagia develops, patients with PD may benefit from changing the food texture and consistency to aid with the eating experience while maintaining the adequate amount of food intake. When patients with PD cannot take in adequate foods orally, tube feedings may be needed.

Parkinson's disease is a dopamine deficient disease that affects movement and coordination. The PD drug, levodopa (L-dopa), is synthesized in the brain into dopamine. It is the most important drug for the management of Parkinson's.

Dietary protein affects L-dopa efficacy; therefore, it is important to modify patients' protein intake to assure adequate protein intake, but not too much. At the same time, we can schedule the eating time an hour after taking L-dopa to minimize the competition between dietary protein and medication. Protein redistribution plan can also be implemented to improve the movement during the day. That is to eat less protein for breakfast and lunch and to eat more protein at dinner and evening.

In summary, a meal plan with protein modification for patients with PD should be developed based on the stages of PD, medical symptoms, individual nutritional needs, culture and personal food preference, daily routines, and lifestyles.

Below is an example of a meal plan for an elderly Chinese woman with Stage Two of PD:

7 am: PD medication

8 am: Breakfast:
- 1 cup rice soup (congee) (½ cup rice, ½ cup water)
- 1 cup mung bean soup (½ cup beans, ½ cup water) (with 1 tbsp. sugar)
- 1 cup stir-fry cabbage (with 1 tbsp. olive oil)
- 1 oz. tofu

11 am: PD medication

Noon: Lunch:
- 1 cup rice
- 1 cup stir-fry Napa cabbage (with 1 tbsp. olive oil)
- 1 cup stir-fry onions with kidney beans (½ cup onions, ½ cup kidney beans, 1 tsp. coconut oil)
- 1 oz. chicken deli slice
- 1 cup strawberries

4 pm: PD medication

5 pm: Dinner:
- 1 cup soy milk
- 3 oz. salmon
- 1 cup stir-fry broccoli (1tbsp. oil)
- 1 cup rice
- ½ cup blueberries

9 pm: PD medication

10 pm: Snack: 1 cup coconut milk

This meal plan has about 1,700 calories, 55 grams of protein, and 70 grams of fats.

Chapter 3: Prepare Healthy Meals for Patients with PD

Meal planning and preparation take some work, but once you learn the skills and get into the habit, you will find that it is worth the effort.

In this chapter, I will show you step-by-step on how to prepare healthy meals for patients with PD. The first step includes some tables and requires some calculations. If you prefer not to make calculations, you can skip the first step, and start with the step 2 (Purchase and Gather all Ingredients).

You can either design your own meals or you can use the ones that I have listed in chapter 4. Designing your own meal plan will give you more flexibility. You can incorporate your culture, food preference, and your creativity into your own meal plan. Let's start with the first step!

Step 1: Design Healthy Meal Plans for Patients with PD

Know Patients' Food Preference and Expand Their Healthy Food Choices

Eating is a very personal event. Everyone has his or her personal food preference.

To help my patients have a meal plan that meets their nutritional needs as well as their culture and personal preference, I always ask my patients to record a 3-day food diary prior to their first nutrition visit with me. I use the food record to discuss their daily eating and food preference. During the nutrition session, I help my patients to develop a list of their food preferences and choices that they are willing to try. I always focus on what they can have instead of what they need to avoid.

There are three purposes of doing this list. First, I use this list as an educational tool. There are ten categories of foods I put on the list. While we are filling out the list, I share some nutritional information and encourage my patients to try certain healthy food items. Second, I will use the list as a base to help them design their meal plan. Third, we will update the list as patients expand their food choices. This is to help them to increase the variety of healthy food choices in their diet.

Below is an example of a patient's food preference and choices that he or she is willing to try:

	Food Preference	Food Choices to Try
Fruit	Banana Strawberries Grapes	Apples Oranges Pears
Vegetables	Potato Iceberg Lettuce Baby carrots	Cucumber Napa Cabbage
Meats	Beef Chicken Pork Sausages	
Seafood	Shrimp	Salmon
Beans		Kidney Beans
Oils & Fats	Corn oil	Olive oil Avocado
Nuts & Seeds	Peanuts	Almonds
Soy Beans		Edamame
Grains	Bread Pasta Pizza Rice	Oat meals Cheerios
Water & Fluid	Water	Tea

Eating Time, Schedule, and Eating Setting

Everyone has his or her own daily routine. Some patients with Parkinson's disease (PD) may have time to eat a healthy breakfast at home while others may need to eat on the go. Some patients may need to reschedule their meal time because they are taking certain medications such as L-dopa.

When designing a meal plan, we usually start with the timings and the settings first. Below is an example of the timings and the settings for a patient with PD:

Timing	Food	Setting
6 am: L-dopa		Home
7 am: Breakfast		Home
10 am: Snack		Work
11 am: L-dopa		Work
Noon: Lunch		Work
4 pm: L-dopa		Home
5 pm: Dinner		Home
8 pm: L-dopa		Home
9 pm: Snack		Home

Estimate Caloric Needs of the Meal

You can use the following two tables from the "Dietary Guidelines 2015-2020" to estimate your caloric needs. The estimated calorie needs are for various age and sex groups at different levels of physical activity. These estimates are based on the Estimated Energy Requirements (EER) equations, using reference heights (average) and reference weights (healthy) for each age-sex group. For adults, the reference man is 5 feet 10 inches tall and weighs 154 pounds. The reference woman is 5 feet 4 inches tall and weighs 126 pounds. Due to reductions in basal metabolic rate that occur with aging, calorie needs generally decrease as we age.

Estimated Daily Calorie Needs for Men, by Age, and Physical Activity Level

Age	Sedentary	Moderately active
21-25	2,400	2,800
26-30	2,400	2,600
31-35	2,400	2,600
36-40	2,400	2,600
41-45	2,200	2,600
46-50	2,200	2,400
51-55	2,200	2,400
56-60	2,200	2,400
61-65	2,000	2,400
66 and up	2,000	2,200

Estimated Daily Calorie Needs for Women, by Age, and Physical Activity Level

Age	Sedentary	Moderately active
21-25	2,000	2,200
26-30	1,800	2,000
31-35	1,800	2,000
36-40	1,800	2,000
41-45	1,800	2,000
46-50	1,800	2,000
51-55	1,600	1,800
56-60	1,600	1,800
61-65	1,600	1,800
66 and up	1,600	1,800

Using the two tables above, you can find the estimated daily caloric needs. As noted in the previous chapter, dinner is usually bigger than breakfast and lunch because more than half of the daily protein will be provided at dinner and evening.

Below is an example of how to estimate the caloric needs of meals and snacks for a 65 year old woman:

By using the table above, the estimated needs for a 65 year old woman with sedentary lifestyle is 1,600 calories a day. Considering her daily routine and her personal preference, she will have three meals and one snack. Since dinner will be her biggest meal of the day, her estimated caloric needs for breakfast and lunch will be 300-500 calories each; her estimated caloric needs for dinner will be 500-600 calories; and her estimated caloric needs for the snack will be 100-200 calories. We will need to monitor her weight to assure that the meal plan provides adequate calories. If the patient starts to lose weight with the meal plan, we will need to adjust up the meal plan and to increase the daily total calories to prevent further weight loss.

Know Their Appetite

Appetite differs among people. Appetite also changes as a result of aging, medication, physical activities, and medical condition. It is important to know patients' appetite when we help them to develop their meal plan. For patients who have bigger appetite and can easily eat 3-5 cups of food per meal, incorporate lots of healthy low caloric density foods such as fruits and vegetables will be a good idea. On the other hand, for patients who have a small appetite and can only eat 1-2 cups of food per meal, choosing higher caloric density foods will be necessary in order to meet their daily caloric needs. Patients with smaller appetite may also benefit from having more snacks in addition to their three meals.

Is There Any Eating or Swallowing Difficulties?

When individuals have difficulty chewing, eating and/or swallowing, it is critical to create menus that meet their nutritional needs while considering these challenges.

Commercial food thickeners, such as Thick-It and Thick and Easy, can help to improve patients' eating experience and total food intake. These products can be used to achieve desired consistency in pureed foods and beverages. Different amount of these products can be used to achieve three different food consistencies: Nectar Consistency, Honey Consistency, and Pudding Consistency. The products usually are easily dissolves in cold and hot drinks. And they do not change the taste or appearance of hot or cold pureed foods and beverages.

Many of the original thickening products contain starch (carbohydrates), so they may not be appropriate for patients who have diabetes. Patients with PD need to consult their physician or feeding therapists before starting the food thickeners. In addition, their meal plan need to be modified since adding food thickeners also increases the total amount of carbohydrates and calories of the meal.

How Much Fat in One Meal?

Fats are essential nutrients and they are very important for the health of your brain. After estimating the caloric needs of the meal, let's move on to estimate the appropriate amount of fats for the meal.

Before I show you how to estimate the fat amount for the meal, let's review some basic nutrition information on energy, i.e. calories. Three major nutrients provide energy which we need for the daily function. They are fats, carbohydrates, and protein. One gram of dietary fat equals nine calories; one gram of carbohydrate provides four calories; and one gram of protein is equal to four calories.

As noted earlier in this book, I suggest that 35% calories come from fats. Based on this, let's calculate the amount of fats needed for a meal. For a breakfast containing 400 calories, the estimated fat amount is calculated as followed:

$400 \times 35\% = 140$ (calories)

One gram fat provides 9 calories.

$140 \div 9 = 15$ (grams)

15 grams of fats is about 1 tbsp. oil or fats.

The following breakfast has about 1 tbsp. good fats from ½ large avocado.

- 1 bean avocado burrito (½ cup bean, ½ large avocado, 1 wrap)
- 1 apple

How Much Protein in One Meal?

Dietary proteins are essential nutrients for our health. They are large, complex molecules that play many critical functions in our body. Proteins are made up of many of smaller units called amino acids. Proteins are needed for all aspects of our body structures and functions such as organs, tissues, hormones, and enzymes.

There are two ways to estimate your protein needs. First, you can use the table below to estimate the daily protein needs.

Daily Protein Recommendations for Adult Men and Women

Protein/Gender	Adult Men	Adult Women
Protein (g)	56	46
Protein % calories	10-35%	10-35%

Source: Dietary Guidelines 2015-2020 Recommendations and Institute of Medicine. Dietary Reference Intakes: The essential guide to nutrient requirements. Washington (DC): The National Academies Press; 2006.

Second, you can estimate your protein needs based on your body weight. The recommended daily protein amount is 0.8 grams per kilogram of body weight. The elderly patients with PD may need more than current Recommended Dietary Allowance (RDA) to maintain physical function and optimal health.

When I work with patients with PD, I usually start with 0.8 g/kg body weight while monitoring their weight.

For example, a man with a body weight of 180 lbs., his RDA for protein will be 66 grams per day. This is how I calculate it:

180 lb. divided by 2.2 equals to 82 kilograms.

82 kilograms multiply by 0.8 equals to 66 grams per day.

To reduce the dietary protein and L-dopa competition during the day, this patient will have more than half of his protein at dinner and evening. This is how I estimate his protein needs for the meals and snacks:

- Breakfast: 10 grams protein
- Lunch: 10 grams protein
- Afternoon snack: no protein
- Dinner: 40 grams protein
- Evening snack: 6 grams protein

You can use the following table, Protein Contents of Common Foods, to design a meal plan that meets your personal preference.

Protein Contents of Common Foods

Item	Amount	Calories	Protein (g)
Chicken breast	3 oz.	150	26
Roast beef	3 oz.	160	24
Pork chop	3 oz.	150	24
Salmon	3 oz.	120	23
Ground beef	3 oz.	200	22
Egg	One	80	8
Kidney beans	½ cup	100	8
Mung beans	½ cup	100	8
Soy milk	1 cup	100	8
Tofu (soft-firm)	3 oz.	70	7
Quinoa	½ cup	100	4
Almonds (nuts)	2 tbsp.	100	4
Almond butter	1 tbsp.	100	4
Hemp seed	1 tbsp.	60	3
Sunflower seeds	2 tbsp.	100	3

Peas	½ cup	50	3
Pasta	½ cup cooked	100	3
Rice (grains)	½ cup cooked	100	2
Sweet potatoes	½ cup cooked	100	2
Mung bean sprouts	½ cup cooked	12	1.5
Almond milk	1 cup	30-90	1-2
Squash	½ cup cooked	30	1
Broccoli	½ cup	15	1
mushrooms	½ cup raw	8	1

Note: These are approximate numbers.

Here is one healthy breakfast with 10 grams of protein:

- 1 bean avocado burrito (½ cup bean, ½ avocado, 1 wrap)
- 1 apple

Weight loss is a common concern among patients with PD. If a patient with PD has failed to maintain his or her body weight and/or lean muscle mass with 0.8 g/kg body weight, I will increase the dietary protein to 1.0 g/kg body weight.

How Much Dietary Fiber in One Meal?

Dietary fibers increase the bioavailability of L-dopa, thus improve patients' motor function. It also helps to prevent constipation which is a common problem among people with Parkinson's.

Daily Adequate Intake for Fiber Set by the Institute of Medicine: 14 Grams per 1,000 Calories

For most adults, this translates to 28-35 grams a day.

This is how I will estimate the dietary fiber needs of the meals and snacks for patients with Parkinson's:

Each meal will have at least 5 grams of dietary fiber. The goal is to have about 10 grams of dietary fiber each meal.

The snack will provide 0-5 grams dietary fiber.

The following breakfast has about 10 grams of dietary fiber:

- 1 cup oatmeal cooked (in water, 1-2 tsp. sugar to taste)
- ½ cup blueberries
- 1 cup coconut milk (This is a milk substitute, not the can version. The canned one is very high in fats and is usually used for cooking or for baking.)
- 6 almonds
- ½ avocado

Carbohydrates are essential building blocks for our body including our genes such as deoxyribonucleic acid or DNA. In addition, carbohydrates are one of the major energy sources for our body. Many of our organs such as the brain and the red blood cells use glucose as a major energy source. This explains the reason why some people on a low-carb diet may experience light headedness, fatigue, and headaches.

Studies have found that diets with stable higher carbs to protein ratios such as 5:1 or 7:1 have improved motor functions. These findings indicated that a stringent daytime protein restriction (less than 7 grams) is not necessary. In addition, an approach like this allows more protein intake during daytime and it is much easier for patients with PD to comply with than the protein restricted diet.

Carbohydrate Contents of Common Foods

Items/Carb amount	15 grams	30 grams	45 grams
Grains			
Bread (slice)	1 slice	2 slices	
Bagel			1
Burger bun	½	1	
Breakfast Cereals	½ -1 cup		
Pizza (large)		1 slice	
Pizza (medium)	1 slice	2 slices	
Pasta	½ cup	1 cup	1 ½ cups
Rice	½ cup	1 cup	1 ½ cups
Starchy Veggies			
Beans	½ cup	1 cup	
Potato (medium)	½	1	
Sweet potato (medium)	½	1	
Squash	1 cup	2 cups	
Dairy			
Milk	1 cup		
Ice cream	½ cup	1cup	
Fruits			
Apple (small)	1		
Banana (medium)	½	1	
Grapes	1 cup		

Please note that these are approximate numbers for easy calculations; therefore, you can apply the information on a daily basis.

Below are three steps that I use to estimate the percentage of carbs for patients with Parkinson's disease:

- First, as noted earlier, I recommend that 35% calories come from fats.
- Second, about 12% calories come from protein.
- Third, subtract fat and protein percentages from total % calories to yield the percentage of carbs. That is 100% - 35% - 12% = 53%. The answer will be 53% carb calories.

Now let's apply this number and do a practice. For a 60 years old woman with sedentary lifestyle, based on the 2015-2020 Dietary Guidelines, she will need 1,600 calories a day.

Since 53% calories will come from carbs, her daily carbs needs will be 212 grams. This is how I make the calculations:

1,600 calories × 53% = 848 calories (from carbs)

One gram carbohydrate equals to 4 calories.

848 ÷ 4 = 212 (grams)

Since her meal plan consists of three meals and one snack, each meal will need 60-70 grams carbs. The following lunch has about 60 grams of carbs:

- 2 cups pasta (1½ cups pasta noodle, ½ cup pasta sauce, 5 tsp. olive oil)
- 1 orange

Step 2: Purchase and Gather all Ingredients

As a dietitian, one of the questions that I have been asked often is what to buy. Cooking healthy meals is much easier when you keep your kitchen stocked with the following ingredients:

- Olive oil
- Coconut oil
- Sesame oil
- Salt
- Black pepper
- Vinegar
- Brown sugar
- Honey
- Maple syrup
- Coconut milk
- Dried kidney beans
- Dried mung beans
- Rice
- Pasta
- Oats
- Almonds, cashews, pistachio nuts, walnuts
- Peanut butter and/or almond butter
- Seaweed
- Coffee or tea
- Frozen corns
- Frozen peas
- Frozen Edamame

When I do my weekly shopping, I always make sure I purchase the following items:

- Eggs
- Tofu
- Meats
- Fish
- Bread
- Uncured deli meats
- Avocados
- Garlics, gingers, green onions
- Cabbage
- Broccoli
- Napa cabbage
- Celery
- Carrots
- Onions
- Cucumbers
- Beets
- Mushrooms
- 1-2 green leafy vegetables
- Lemons
- Apples
- Oranges
- Banana
- Pears
- Berries if in season

Once you have purchased and gathered all the ingredients you need, you can start trying the recipes that I have included in this book.

Step 3: Measure and Weigh the Ingredients and Portion Sizes

Using kitchen measuring tools, you can cook and serve the right portion size for the meals and snacks that you have developed.

I recommend that you purchase the following measuring tools:

- Stainless steel measuring cups and spoons
- Kitchen digital measuring scales

Common Measurement Conversions

Cup	Fluid oz.	TBSP.	TSP.
1 cup	8 fl. oz.	16 tbsp.	48 tsp.
½ cup	4 fl. oz.	8 tbsp.	24 tsp.
¼ cup	2 fl. oz.	4 tbsp.	12 tsp.

Chapter 4: Healthy Meals and Snacks for Patients with PD

I have written the following 14 meals and 14 snacks, structured to provide the proper number of servings as recommended in chapter 3. Each of the healthy foods mentioned in this book has been incorporated into the meals and snacks at least once. You can mix and match these meals and snacks to make your own weekly menu. In addition, I have included recipes in the second part of this chapter.

14 Healthy Breakfasts for Patients with PD

Below are fourteen healthy breakfasts. Each breakfast contains 10 grams or less protein. This will help to maximize L-dopa effects and ameliorate motor function during daytime. These meals are rich in dietary fibers, good fats, vitamins, minerals, and phytonutrients.

Healthy Breakfast #1:
- 1 cup oatmeal cooked (in water, 1-2 tsp. sugar to taste)
- ½ cup blueberries
- 1 cup coconut milk (This is a milk substitute, not the can version. The canned one is very high in fats and is usually used for cooking or for baking.)
- 6 almonds
- ½ avocado

Healthy Breakfast #2:

- Coconut Milkshake (See recipe #1 on page 84.)
  (This milkshake has ½ avocado, 1 banana, ½ cup
  strawberries, 1 cup coconut milk, and 1-3 tsp. sugar
  to taste.)

Healthy Breakfast #3:

- 1 cup dark coffee (If you like, you can add some
  coconut milk and/or sugar.)
- 6 crackers
- ½ medium avocado
- 1 cup grapes
- 12 almonds

Healthy Breakfast #4:

- 1 cup Cheerios
- 1 cup almond milk
- 1 orange
- 6 almonds

Healthy Breakfast #5 (Chinese dishes):

- 1 cup rice soup (congee) (½ cup rice, ½ cup water)
- 1 cup mung bean soup (½ cup beans, ½ cup water)
  (with 1 tbsp. sugar(optional))
- 1 cup stir-fry cabbage (with 1 tbsp. olive oil)
- 1 oz. tofu with 1 tsp. soy sauce

Healthy Breakfast #6 (Indian dishes):

- 2-3 rice bun (cake)
- 4 tbsp. bean curry
- 1 cup coconut milk

71

Healthy Breakfast #7:

- 1 cup mung bean soup (½ cup bean, ½ cup water, 1 tbsp. sugar)
- 1 avocado
- 1 orange

Healthy Breakfast #8:

- 1 cup coconut rice pudding (See recipe #2 on page 85.)
- ½ cup blueberries
- 6 cashews
- 1 cup dark coffee (If you like, you can add some coconut milk and/or sugar.)

Healthy Breakfast #9:

- 1 bean avocado burrito (½ cup bean, ½ avocado, 1 wrap)
- 1 apple
- 1 cup green tea

Healthy Breakfast #10:

- 1 peanut butter sandwiches (2 whole wheat bread, 1 tbsp. peanut butter, 1 tbsp. strawberry jelly)
- 1 cup coconut milk
- 1 orange

Healthy Breakfast #11:

- 1 cup hot millet porridge with cinnamon and nutmeg (½ cup cooked millet)
- 1 cup blueberries or raspberries

- 1 tablespoon pecans
- ½ cup or 1 oz. coconut chips
- 1 cup coffee

Healthy Breakfast #12:
- 1 pancake
- 1 tbsp. coconut oil
- 1 tbsp. maple syrup
- 1 cup cut strawberries
- 1 cup coffee

Healthy Breakfast #13:
- 1 waffle
- 1 tbsp. coconut oil
- 1 tbsp. maple syrup
- 1 cup cut strawberries
- 1 cup coffee

Healthy Breakfast #14 (Chinese dishes):
- 1 green onion bun
- 1 green tea
- 1 orange
- 1 avocado

14 Healthy Lunches for Patients with PD

Below are fourteen healthy lunches. Each lunch contains 10 grams or less protein. This will help to ameliorate motor function during daytime. These meals are rich in dietary fibers, good fats, vitamins, minerals, and phytonutrients.

Healthy Lunch #1:
- 1 cup rice
- 1 cup stir-fry Napa cabbage (with 1 tbsp. olive oil)
- 1 cup stir-fry onions with kidney beans (½ cup onions, ½ cup kidney beans, 1 tsp. coconut oil)
- 1 cup strawberries
- 1 cup black tea

Healthy Lunch #2 (Mexican dishes):
- 1 bean avocado burrito (½ cup bean, ½ avocado, 1 wrap)
- 1 cup salad (lettuce, tomato, carrots) with 1 tbsp. dressing
- 1 cup strawberries

Healthy Lunch #3 (Japanese dishes):
- 1 avocado sushi roll (6 pieces)
- 1 cup miso soup
- 1 apple

Healthy Lunch #4 (Japanese dishes):
- 1 California sushi roll (6 pieces)
- 1 apple
- 1 coconut milk

Healthy Lunch #5:

- 1 peanut butter sandwiches (2 whole wheat bread, 1 tbsp. peanut butter, 1 tbsp. strawberry jelly)
- ½ cup or 1 oz. coconut chips
- 1 apple
- 1 cup dark coffee (If you like, you can add some coconut milk and/or sugar.)

Healthy Lunch #6:

- 2 cups pasta (1½ cups pasta noodle, ½ cup pasta sauce, 5 tsp. olive oil)
- 1 orange
- 1 cup dark coffee (If you like, you can add some coconut milk and/or sugar.)

Healthy Lunch #7:

- 3 cups salad (2 cups lettuce, ½ tomato, 10 olives, ½ avocado, ½ cup beets, 6 cashews) with 1-2 tbsp. dressing
- 1 dinner roll
- 1 cup green tea

Healthy Lunch #8:

- 1 corn tortilla
- ½ cup hummus
- 1 cup grapes
- 1 cup dark coffee (If you like, you can add some coconut milk and/or sugar.)
- ½ cup or 1 oz. coconut chips

Healthy Lunch #9 (Chinese dishes):

- 2 cups vegetable stir-fry rice (See recipe #10 on page 93)
- 1 cup green tea
- 1 orange

Healthy Lunch #10:

- Coconut Milkshake (See recipe #1 on page 84.) (This milkshake has ½ avocado, 1 banana, ½ cup strawberries, 1 cup coconut milk, and 1-3 tsp. sugar to taste.)

Healthy Lunch #11: (Thai dishes)

- 1 cup Thai coconut curry soup with vegetables and garbanzo beans
- ½ cup brown rice
- 1 cup green tea with lemon
- 1 orange

Healthy Lunch #12:

- 1 cup tomato-basil soup
- 6 whole-grain crackers
- 1 avocado
- 1 cup black tea
- 1 apple

Healthy Lunch #13:

- Hummus sandwich (2 bread, ¼ cup hummus, tomato, ½ avocado, spinach)
- 1 cup black coffee
- 1 pear

Healthy Lunch #14 (Chinese dishes):

- 1 cup hot and sour soup
- 1 ½ cups vegetable stir-fry rice (See recipe #10 on page 93.)
- 1 cup green tea
- 1 apple

14 Healthy Dinners for Patients with PD

Below are fourteen healthy dinners that contain plenty of protein, dietary fibers, good fats, vitamins, minerals, and phytonutrients. These dinners contain 30 grams or more of protein. One of these dinners alone meets half or more than half of daily protein needs for many of the patients with Parkinson's disease.

Healthy Dinner #1:
- 1 cup soy milk
- 3 oz. pan-fry salmon
- 1 cup stir-fry broccoli (1tbsp. oil)
- 1 ½ cups rice
- ½ cup blueberries

Healthy Dinner #2:
- 1 medium sweet potato
- 6 oz. salmon
- 1 cup spinach
- 1 tbsp. olive oil

Healthy Dinner #3:
- 1 ½ cups brown rice
- 6 oz. tofu
- 1 boiled egg
- 12 cashews
- 1 cup broccoli
- 1 tbsp. olive oil for cooking

Healthy Dinner #4:
- 1 cup brown rice
- 1 cup cooked kidney beans
- 1 cup green beans with ground pork (1-2 cups green beans, 1 oz. ground pork) (See recipe #7 on page 90.)
- 1 tbsp. olive oil

Healthy Dinner #5:
- 1 cup soy milk
- 3 oz. salmon
- 2 cups salad with 2 tbsp. dressing
- 1 medium potato
- ½ cup blueberries

Healthy Dinner #6:
- 1 peanut butter sandwich (2 slice bread, 3 tbsp. peanut butter, 1 tbsp. strawberry jelly)
- 1 cup soy milk
- ½ cup baby carrots

Healthy Dinner #7 (Indian dishes):
- 2 Chapatti
- 1 cup lentil curry with 1 tbsp. coconut oil
- ½ cooked beet root
- 2 oz. fish

Healthy Dinner #8:
- 2 cups chicken noodle soup (1 cup noodle, ½ cup chicken, 2 tsp. olive oil)
- 1 side salad with 1-2 tbsp. dressing
- 1 oz. dark chocolate

Healthy Dinner #9 (Chinese dishes):
- 2 cups vegetable stir-fry rice (See recipe #10 on page 93.)
- 3 oz. pan-fry cod fish.
- 1 cup soy milk

Healthy Dinner #10 (Chinese dishes):
- 2 ½ cups egg stir-fry rice (See recipe #3 on page 86.)(1 ½ cups rice, ½ cup corn, ½ cup peas, 2 eggs, 2 oz. ham, 2 tbsp. olive oil, 1 tbsp. sesame oil, salt, spices to taste)
- 1 cup coconut milk

Healthy Dinner #11:
- 1 cup split pea soup
- 1 dinner roll
- 1 oz. dark chocolate
- 1 cup green tea

Healthy Dinner #12:
- Scrambled eggs (2 eggs, 1 tbsp. coconut oil, salt)
- 1 sweet potato
- 1 cup strawberries
- 1 black tea

Healthy Dinner #13:
- 3-5 oz. sea bass
- 1 cup winter squash
- 1 cup stir-fry broccoli (1 cup broccoli, 1 tbsp. coconut oil)
- 1 cup soy milk

Healthy Dinner #14 (Mexican dishes):
- 2 fish tacos (2 taco shells, 3-5 oz. fish, ½ cup cabbage and carrots, ½ cup beans)
- ¼ cup salsa
- 1 apple

14 Healthy Snacks for Patients with PD

Below are fourteen healthy snacks for patients with Parkinson's disease. These snacks contain minimum protein and will not significantly affect the efficacy of L-dopa. These snacks are rich in one or more of the following nutrients: dietary fibers, good fats, vitamins, minerals or phytonutrients.

Healthy Snack #1: 1-2 cups fresh fruit

Healthy Snack #2: 1 cup coconut milk

Healthy Snack #3: 1 small avocado

Healthy Snack #4: ¼ cup banana chips (ingredients: banana, coconut oil, fruit juice)

Healthy Snack #5: 8-16 oz. coconut water

Healthy Snack #6: 4-8 oz. 100% fruit juice

Healthy Snack #7: ½ cup raw vegetables such as baby carrots or celery stick or cucumber

Healthy Snack #8: 4-6 olives

Healthy Snack #9: ½ cup beets

Healthy Snack #10: 1 oz. or ½ cup coconut chips

Healthy Snack #11: 1 cup coffee (with sugar &/or coconut milk)

Healthy Snack: #12: 1 cup lemonade

Healthy Snack #13: 1 cup black tea (with sugar &/or coconut milk)

Healthy Snack #14: 1 cup pickled cucumber (See recipe #6 on page 89.)

Recipe

1. Coconut Milkshake

- Put ½ avocados in the blender.
- Add one chopped banana to the blender.
- Add ½ cup strawberries.
- Put 1 cup coconut milk (milk substitute, not the one from the can).
- Add 1-3 tsp. sugar to taste.
- Blender them together and serve it as a healthy breakfast or lunch.

2. Coconut Rice Pudding

- Cook 1 cup coconut milk and ½ cup rice in a saucepan at low heat.
- Add 1 tbsp. brown sugar, a little cinnamon, and vanilla.
- Add 1 tbsp. coconut oil and mix it thoroughly.
- Cook it at low heat for few minutes until rice is soft.
- You can serve it hot or put it in the fringe and cool it for 30-60 minutes.
- Serve this coconut rice pudding with ½ cup blueberries and 6 cashews for a healthy breakfast.

3. Egg Stir-Fry Rice

- Cook rice in a rice cooker following the instructions on the rice cooker.
- Chop some green onions and set aside.
- Dice up 2 oz. uncured ham and set aside.
- Heat 2 tbsp. olive oil in the pan for 30 seconds.
- Add chopped green onions and salt to taste.
- Add ½ cup frozen peas and ½ cup frozen corns to the pan. Stir them well and cook them at medium heat until peas and corns are hot.
- Add 1 ½ cups of cooked rice to the pan. Add 1 tbsp. sesame oil and some salt and soy sauce to taste.
- Crack two eggs to the bowel and lightly beat it. Add a little salt to the eggs.
- Add the eggs to the vegetables and rice in the pan. Stir fry it at medium heat for 3-5 minutes until the eggs are cooked.
- Add the diced 2 oz. ham to the pan and mix it well.
- Serve this as a healthy dinner. I personally love to put some seaweed on top of the stir-fry rice. They go very well together.

4. Indian fish and coconut stew

- Heat 1 tbsp. olive oil in a pan.
- Add seeds and spices for 1 minute.
- Add the chopped onions and a little salt to taste and cook for 10 minutes.
- Add ½ cup coconut milk and mix it well.
- Add 3 oz. cod fish to the pan.
- Cover and cook at the low to medium heat for 10 minutes.
- Serve it with 1 cup rice and 1 cup broccoli for a healthy dinner.

- Add a little salt to cover 6 oz. salmon.
- Add 1 tbsp. flour to cover the salmon with very thin layer (This will prevent the fish to break.)
- Heat 1 tbsp. olive oil in the pan.
- Add the fish to the pan and cover it for 3 minutes.
- Flip the fish and cover it for another 3 minutes.
- Serve it with 1 medium potato and a side salad for a healthy dinner.

6. Pickled Cucumber

- If you use English cucumber or Persian cucumber, you don't need to take out the seeds.
- If you use regular cucumber, slice it in the middle and take out the seeds.
- Chop the cucumber into slices.
- Add 2 tbsp. extra virgin olive oil or sesame oil to the sliced cucumber.
- Add 1 tbsp. vinegar to the cucumber.
- Add a little salt to taste.
- Mix them well and serve.
- You can save this pickled cucumber in the fringe for up to a week.
- You can serve a cup of pickle cucumber as part of a healthy meal.

- Season 1 oz. ground pork with salt and black pepper.

- Smashed and chopped some garlic.
- Heat 1 tbsp. olive oil in the pot.
- Add the chopped garlic and ground pork to the pot and cook for 3-5 minutes at medium heat.
- Add 2 cup green beans to the pot.
- Add 2 tsp. olive oil to the pot.
- Add a little salt and white pepper to the pot and mix it well.
- Cover it for 1-2 minutes. Stir it a few times to prevent it from burning. Add 1-3 tbsp. water as needed. Repeat this for few times until green beans are cooked.
- You can serve this with 1 cup of rice for a healthy lunch.
- You can also serve this with 1 cup of rice and 2 scrambled eggs for a healthy dinner.

- Rinse the Napa cabbage and cut it the middle.
- Put half of the Napa cabbage back in the refrigerator for next time usage.
- Chop the Napa cabbage into pieces.
- Heat 2 tbsp. olive oil in the pan.
- Add chopped garlic and a little bit of salt to the pan.
- Add the chopped Napa cabbage to the pan.
- Cover it and cook it at medium heat for 3-5 minutes. Stir it every minute to prevent it from burning. Add 1-3 tbsp. water as needed.
- Enjoy a cup of stir-fry Napa cabbage as part of your healthy lunch or dinner.

9. **Stir-Fry Onion and Kidney Beans**

- Heat 1 tbsp. olive oil in the pot.
- Add the chopped onions to the pot and cook for 5 minutes at medium heat.
- Add a little salt to taste.
- Add 1 cup cooked kidney beans to the pot. (It's best to soak and cook the beans ahead of time or you can use the can beans. Store the unused cooked beans in a separate glass container and save it in the freezer for later usage.)
- Add 2 tsp. olive oil to the pot.
- Add a little salt and white pepper to the pot and mix it well. (If you use the can one, you may not need to add salt. Many of the can beans have added salt already.)
- Cover it for 1-2 minutes. Stir it to prevent it from burning. Repeat this for few times until kidney beans are soft.
- You can serve this with 1 cup of rice for a healthy lunch.
- You can also serve this with 1 cup of rice or one tortilla wrap and some baby carrots for a healthy dinner.

10. Vegetable Stir-Fry Rice

- Cook rice in a rice cooker following the instructions on the rice cooker.
- Chop some green onions and set aside.
- Heat 2 tbsp. olive oil in the pan for 30 seconds.
- Add chopped green onions and salt to taste.
- Add ½ cup frozen peas and ½ cup frozen corns to the pan. Stir them well and cook them at medium heat until peas and corns are hot.
- Add 1 ½ cups of cooked rice to the pan. Add 1 tbsp. sesame oil and some salt and soy sauce to taste.
- You can serve this dish as a healthy lunch. Personally I love to put some seaweed on top of the stir-fry rice. They go very well together.
- You can also serve the stir-fry rice with 3 oz. pan-fry salmon for a healthy dinner.

- Add 1 tbsp. extra virgin olive oil to 1 cup salad. Toss it lightly to coat the vegetables with olive oil. Olive oil will help the absorption of nutrients from the vegetables.
- Add 1 tsp. vinegar.
- Add some black pepper and salt to taste.

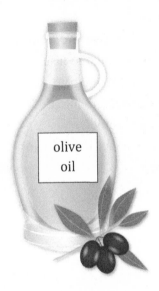

12. Mung Bean Soup

Compared to most beans, mung beans take shorter time to cook. Here are the steps that I take to cook mung bean soup:

- I purchase dry whole mung beans.
- Soak mung beans in water overnight.
- Rinse mung beans several times until the water is clean and clear.
- I use Tatung Rice cooker to cook mung beans. This rice cooker uses indirect heat like a steamer. I put twice amount of water to cover mung beans. In the outer pot of the rice cooker, I use 6 oz. water to boil and steam mung bean soup. It will take about 30 minutes to cook the beans.
- Once it's cooked, you can take out one cup of mung bean soup (½ cup mung bean, ½ cup water) and add one tbsp. sugar to become a sweet soup. You can serve this with an avocado for a healthy breakfast.
- When I grew up in Taiwan, my mom cooked rice with mung bean to become rice mung bean soup (without sugar). We ate the rice mung bean soup with separate dishes of vegetables and tofu as a healthy breakfast. You can have 1 ½ cups soup (½ cup mung bean, ¼ cup rice, remaining water), 1 cup stir-fry cabbage (1 tbsp. olive oil), 1 oz. tofu & 20 peanuts for a healthy breakfast.

Chapter 5: Summary

Parkinson's disease (PD) is a progressive disease. The motor progression and fluctuation can be challenging. As noted earlier in this book, patients with PD can benefit from certain dietary interventions.

The dietary suggestions and meal plans covered in this book are based on current study findings and my personal clinical judgment for patients with PD. It is my hope that you can use this book as a reference book to manage Parkinson's disease with diet.

The meal plan and recipes listed in this book should not be used for patients with diabetes due to the high carbohydrate contents of the meals and recipes. You need to consult your physician before starting with any treatment plans including dietary suggestions provided in this book.

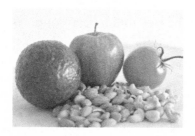

Nutrition Websites

Below is a list of websites that may be of interest to you:

Academy of Nutrition and Dietetics
www.eatright.org
This website offers many helpful nutrition resources and information to providers and consumers.

Body Mass Index (BMI) Calculators
www.cdc.gov
On the website, type BMI calculator, it will take you to the page that you can calculate BMI for adults, children, and teens.

Nutrition.gov
www.nutrition.gov
This website provides current dietary recommendations.

Dietary Guidelines 2015-2020
https://health.gov/dietaryguidelines/2015/guidelines/appendix-2/

What to Buy
http://anutritioncounseling.com/home/managing_parkinsons_with_diet
On this website page, you will find the author's personal suggestions on specific food items, supplements, food measurement tools, and kitchenware for patients with Parkinson's disease.

Appendices

Appendix A: Estimated Daily Calorie Needs for Men, by Age, and Physical Activity Level

Age	Sedentary	Moderately Active
21-25	2,400	2,800
26-30	2,400	2,600
31-35	2,400	2,600
36-40	2,400	2,600
41-45	2,200	2,600
46-50	2,200	2,400
51-55	2,200	2,400
56-60	2,200	2,400
61-65	2,000	2,400
66 and up	2,000	2,200

Appendix B: Estimated Daily Calorie Needs for Women, by Age, and Physical Activity Level

Age	Sedentary	Moderately Active
21-25	2,000	2,200
26-30	1,800	2,000
31-35	1,800	2,000
36-40	1,800	2,000
41-45	1,800	2,000
46-50	1,800	2,000
51-55	1,600	1,800
56-60	1,600	1,800
61-65	1,600	1,800
66 and up	1,600	1,800

Items/Fat amount	1 tsp. fat*	2 tsp.*	3 tsp.*
Olive oil	1 tsp.		
Butter or mayo	½ tbsp.	1 tbsp.	
Dressing or cream cheese or gravy or coconut milk	1 tbsp.	2 tbsp.	3 tbsp.
Cheese (1 oz. part skim = 1 fat)	1 oz. feta	1 oz. cheddar	
Avocado (large)	1/6	1/3	½
Peanut butter	2/3 tbsp.		2 tbsp.
Almonds	1 tbsp.	2 tbsp.	3 tbsp.
Guacamole	2 tbsp.	4 tbsp.	8 tbsp.
Bacon	1 slice	2 slices	
Hummus	4 tbsp.	8 tbsp.	12 tbsp.
Salmon	3 oz.	6 oz.	
Ground beef (90% lean)		3 oz.	
Ground beef (80% lean)			3 oz.
Pork chops		3-4 oz.	
Egg (large)	1	2	
Olives (large)	8 olives		
2% milk	1 cup	2 cups	

*Please note that these are approximate numbers for easy calculations; therefore, you can apply the information on a daily basis. For more precise numbers, please visit the USDA National Nutrient Database.

Appendix D: Daily Protein Recommendations for Adult Men and Women

Age/Gender	Adult Men	Adult Women
Protein (g)	56	46
Protein % calories	10-35%	10-35%

Source: Dietary Guidelines 2015-2020 Recommendations and Institute of Medicine. Dietary Reference Intakes: The essential guide to nutrient requirements. Washington (DC): The National Academies Press; 2006.

Appendix E: Protein Contents of Common Foods

Item	Amount	Calories	Protein (g)
Chicken breast	3 oz.	150	26
Roast beef	3 oz.	160	24
Pork chop	3 oz.	150	24
Salmon	3 oz.	120	23
Ground beef	3 oz.	200	22
Egg	One	80	8
Kidney beans	½ cup	100	8
Mung beans	½ cup	100	8
Soy milk	1 cup	100	8
Tofu (soft-firm)	3 oz.	70	7
Quinoa	½ cup	100	4
Almonds (nuts)	2 tbsp.	100	4
Almond butter	1 tbsp.	100	4
Hemp seed	1 tbsp.	60	3
Sunflower seeds	2 tbsp.	100	3
Peas	½ cup	50	3
Pasta	½ cup cooked	100	3
Rice (grains)	½ cup cooked	100	2

Sweet potatoes	½ cup cooked	100	2
Mung bean sprouts	½ cup cooked	12	1.5
Almond milk	1 cup	30-90	1-2
Squash	½ cup cooked	30	1
Broccoli	½ cup	15	1
mushrooms	½ cup raw	8	1

Note: These are approximate numbers.

Appendix F: Dietary Fiber Contents of Common Foods

Food	Portion Size	Fiber per Portion (g)*
Beans (black, kidney)	½ cup cooked	6–9
Green peas, cooked	½ cup	4
Whole-wheat English muffin	1 muffin	4
Raspberries, blackberries	½ cup	4
Sweet potato with skin	1 medium	4
Shredded wheat cereal	1 oz.	4
Avocado	½ medium	4
Apple or pear with skin	1 small	4
Greens (spinach), cooked	½ cup	3
Nuts (Almonds)	1 ounce	3
Whole wheat spaghetti	½ cup cooked	3
Banana	1 medium	3
Orange	1 medium	3
Potato with skin	1 small	3
Winter squash, cooked	½ cup	3
Tomato paste	¼ cup	3
Broccoli, cooked	½ cup	3
Quinoa	½ cup	2.5
Brown Rice	½ cup	2
Strawberries	½ cup	2
Grapes, red or green	½ cup	1

*Please note that these are approximate numbers for easy calculations. For more precise numbers, please visit the USDA National Nutrient Database.

Use the form below to see how much dietary fiber in your diet.

Meals & Snacks	Food Items	Fiber (grams)
Breakfast		
Lunch		
Dinner		
Snack 1		
Snack 2		
Snack 3		
Total		

Appendix H: Carbohydrate Contents of Common Foods

Items/Carb amount	15 grams	30 grams	45 grams
Grains			
Bread (slice)	1 slice	2 slices	
Bagel			1
Burger bun	½	1	
Breakfast Cereals	½ -1 cup		
Pizza (large)		1 slice	
Pizza (medium)	1 slice	2 slices	
Pasta	½ cup	1 cup	1 ½ cups
Rice	½ cup	1 cup	1 ½ cups
Starchy Veggies			
Beans	½ cup	1 cup	
Potato (medium)	½	1	
Sweet potato (medium)	½	1	
Squash	1 cup	2 cups	
Dairy			
Milk	1 cup		
Ice cream	½ cup	1cup	
Fruits			
Apple (small)	1		
Banana (medium)	½	1	
Grapes	1 cup		

Please note that these are approximate numbers for easy calculations; therefore, you can apply the information on a daily basis.

Glossary

Body Mass Index (BMI): It is a person's weight in kilograms divided by the square of height in meters.

Dietary fiber: Carbohydrates that cannot be digested by human body.

Lignin: A constituent of plant cell walls. It is polymer, but not composed of carbohydrates.

Low-fat diet: A diet that has less than 20% calories from fats and oils.

Monounsaturated fats: Fats that have one double bond.

Omega-3 fatty acids: They are part of polyunsaturated fat group.

Polyunsaturated fats: Oils that have two or more double bonds. They are essential for human body.

Registered dietitians: They are nutrition experts who have been accredited by the Academy of Nutrition and Dietetics.

Saturated fats: Fats that have no double bonds.

Trans fats: They are not common in whole foods, but manufactures make them from oils and add them to many processed foods.

Tube feeding: It is a way of getting your body the nutrition it needs by a feeding tube inserted to the stomach.

References

- Marzena UK, Anna BK, et al. Good and bad sides of diet in Parkinson's disease. Nutrition 29 (2013) 474 -475.

- M.H. Saint-Hilaire. Proportioned Carbohydrate: Protein Diet in the Management of Parkinson's Disease. Parkinson's disease and Quality of Life. 2000.

- Luciana B, Chiara B, et al. Pilot dietary study with normoproteic protein-redistributed plant-food diet and motor performance in patients with Parkinson's disease. Nutritional Neuroscience. 2011.

- Densie Webb. Diet and the Risk of Parkinson's disease. Today's Dietitian April 2013.

- Laurie K. M, Richard, C.L., et al. Role of Diet and Nutritional Supplements in Parkinson's disease Progression. Oxidative Medicine and Cellular Longevity. Vol. 2017, article ID 6405278.

- Keiko Tanaka, Yoshihiro Miyake, et al. Intake of Japanese and Chinese teas reduces risk of Parkinson's disease. Parkinsonism and Related Disorders 17 (2011)

- Erica Cassani, Michela Barichella, et al. Dietary habits in Parkinson's disease: Adherence to

Mediterranean diet. Parkinsonism and Related Disorders 42 (2017).

- Sheyda S, Javad M, et. al. Modulatory role of ketogenic diet on neuroinflmamation: a possible drug naïve strategy to treatment of Parkinson's disease. Advances in Bioscience & Clinical Medicine. ISSN: 2203-1413. Vol. 03.

- Freya Kamel, Samuel M. Goldman, et al. Dietary fat intake, pesticide use, and Parkinson's disease. Parkinsonism and Related Disorders 20 (2014) 82e87.

- Mibel M. Pabon, Jennifer N., et al. A Spirulina-Enhanced Diet Provides Neuroprotection in a-Synuclein Model of Parkinson's Disease. PLOS One. September 2012 | Volume 7

- Luxi Wang, Nian Xiong1 et al, Protein Restricted Diet for Ameliorating Motor Fluctuations in Parkinson's disease. Frontiers in Aging Neuroscience. 2017.

About the Author

Yuchi Yang has been a registered dietitian for more than twenty years. She is a graduate in Nutrition from Taipei Medical University and holds a master degree from the University of Connecticut in Nutritional Science. She had her nutrition internship at the University of California, Los Angeles and Children's Hospital, Los Angeles.

Yuchi Yang, RD enjoys working with people to address their nutritional concerns and questions. She had worked as a clinical dietitian at Children's Hospital, Los Angeles and Gouverneur Hospital in New York City providing nutrition counseling on a wide range of medical diagnoses.

Since 2011, Yuchi Yang, RD has been providing nutrition counseling in Issaquah, Washington serving the Greater Seattle Area. She also provides tele-nutrition consultation through Go-to-Meeting and We Chat. For more information, please visit her website at: www.anutritioncounseling.com.

Made in United States
Orlando, FL
31 January 2023

29270304R10075